THIS NOTEBOOK BELONGS TO:

CPSIA information can be obtained
at www.ICGtesting.com
Printed in the USA
BVHW022035070623
665543BV00010B/210

9 782700 995565